Amadou Fall Lo

Health on Health coverage in Senegal

Amadou Fall Lo

Health on Health coverage in Senegal

ScienciaScripts

Imprint
Any brand names and product names mentioned in this book are subject to trademark, brand or patent protection and are trademarks or registered trademarks of their respective holders. The use of brand names, product names, common names, trade names, product descriptions etc. even without a particular marking in this work is in no way to be construed to mean that such names may be regarded as unrestricted in respect of trademark and brand protection legislation and could thus be used by anyone.

Cover image: www.ingimage.com

This book is a translation from the original published under ISBN 978-613-8-46566-9.

Publisher:
Sciencia Scripts
is a trademark of
Dodo Books Indian Ocean Ltd., member of the OmniScriptum S.R.L Publishing group
str. A.Russo 15, of. 61, Chisinau-2068, Republic of Moldova Europe
Printed at: see last page
ISBN: 978-620-4-13596-0

Acknowledgements

In the name of GOD the Most Gracious, the Most Merciful.

This work is dedicated to my grieving Uncle, may he rest in peace.

My grieving brothers, peace in their souls.

My parents,

To my brothers,

My family,

My friends,

My colleagues

My promotionists...

Alhamdou LILAHI.

Summary

In Senegal, only 20% of the population, made up of the formal sector, is covered by a health insurance system, while the informal sector, which represents more than 80% of the population, is only covered to the extent of 7%. Since then, the priority given to financial accessibility to quality health services has been manifested in the development of Universal Health Coverage (UHC) through the adoption of a Strategic Plan for the Development of Universal Health Coverage (PSD-CMU) in accordance with the Government's desire to reduce inequalities through the revitalization of Mutual Health Insurance (MHI). The objective of our study was to explore the points of view of MOH actors on the operational changes brought about by the implementation of the CMU in the Matam region. This is a qualitative study that used in-depth semi-structured interviews with MOH actors. The results focused mainly on themes such as: commitment to the MOH, training of actors, state subsidy, trust in the MOH, work overload with volunteers, and the benefits of the MOH. In order to achieve the CSU through the revitalization of the MOHs, the optics of the compulsory contribution through new information and communication technologies, the computerization of the management of the MOHs to save time and quality in the procedures on the reimbursement and the subsidy, The respect of the framework agreement between the departmental union of the MOHs and the health structures on the compulsory reference and the portability of the coverage within the department, the training of the managers and the transformation of the community management of the MOHs into a "*community enterprise*" orientation in which everyone would be a shareholder are all alternatives that deserve to be explored by the decision-makers

Keywords Universal Health Coverage - Universal Health Coverage - Financial Protection - Health Financing - Mutual Health Insurance - Mutual Scheme - Matam - Change - Stakeholders' perception - Direct payment - Senegal

Abstract

In Senegal, only 20% of the formal sector population is covered by a health insurance system, while the informal sector represents more than 80% of the population is covered only by 7%. The best solution for accessing affordable quality health services was the development of Universal Health Coverage (UHC) through the adoption of a Strategic Plan for the Development of Universal Health Coverage (PSD-CMU) to the will of the government to reduce inequalities through the revitalization of Community-Based Health Insurance (CBHI). The objective of our study was to explore the views of CBHI's actors on the operational changes brought about by the implementation of the UHC in the Matam region. This is a qualitative study that used extensive semi-directive interviews with CBHI actors. The results focused on topics such as: commitment to CBHI, training of stakeholders, state subsidy, confidence in CBHI, overload of work with volunteerism and profit Confers by CBHI. In order to achieve the UHC through the revitalization of CBHI, the perspective of the compulsory contribution through the new information and communication technologies, the computerization of the management of CBHI to save time and quality in the procedures for reimbursement and subsidy, compliance with the framework agreement between the departmental union of CBHI and health facilities on mandatory reference and portability of coverage within the department, training of managers and the transformation of CBHI management into a "community enterprise" orientation in which everyone is a shareholder are alternatives that deserve to be explored by decision makers.

Keywords Universal Health Coverage - Out-Of-Pocket Payment - Health financing - Community-Based health Insurance - scheme insurance - financial health protection - Matam - Change - Perception of Actors - Out OF Pocket Payment- Senegal.

Table of Contents

List of tables and figures

Introduction

At its 58th session, the World Health Assembly promoted in 2005 the development of more equitable and accessible health financing systems oriented towards the most disadvantaged populations with maximum protection against direct payments4. The Universal Health Coverage (UHC) is essentially based on the equitable accessibility of quality health services and financial protection for users6. Indeed, UHC followed the inadequacies of the 1978 Alma Ata orientation on Primary Health Care (PHC) in the "*Health For All by the Year 2000*" strategy based on universal, accessible and scientifically sound services. The cost of these services should be sustainable by the populations through community participation (CP) in terms of direct cost. In order to operationalize this in Africa, the Bamako Initiative was created in 1987, and it allowed the acceleration of this CP in order to facilitate the access of African populations to PHC5-23. Since then, several types of exemption from direct health-related costs have been tested in most of these countries, but these pose problems of financial sustainability for the already poor governments on the one hand, and overuse of services on the other. In a concern for risk sharing and with a view to moving towards UHC, several other systems of protected contributions have emerged, ranging from the establishment of mutual health insurance (MH), to compulsory and even complementary insurance10.

With this in mind, one of the most common forms of payment for health is direct payment for medicines and services at the point of need, and the poorest countries are the ones that make the most use of this type of financing. According to World Health Organization (WHO) estimates in 2013, 150 million people each year are in financial distress as a result of medical expenses, while 100 million people fall below the poverty line simply because they have to use health services and pay directly for them.11'[14]

A number of empirical studies suggest that financial protection systems such as health insurance improve health status without the insured spending more on health care. Thus, joining a health insurance scheme covering health care expenses prevents these expenses from jeopardizing the individual's budget or forcing him to dip into other expenditure items that could improve his health: such as education, housing or food15.

In 2009, the Council of Ministers of the West African Economic and Monetary Union (UEMOA) defined a mutual insurance company in its regulations as: "*a grouping which, essentially through the contributions of its members, proposes to carry out, in the interest of its members and their dependants, a provident, mutual aid and solidarity action aimed at preventing social risks linked to the person and repairing their consequences*". The mutualist principles also define the characteristic reference values with which a mutual company is identified, in particular

- Voluntary and non-discriminatory membership is a voluntary act of participation in MS not based on gender, race, nationality, political or religious affiliation,

- Non-profit implies that the activities are conducted for a purpose other than making a profit,

- democratic and participatory operation means the participation of members, either directly or through their representatives, in the operation of the institution,

- the commitment to solidarity is based on mutual aid between members with a view to sharing risks,

- autonomy and independence imply the free administration of the institution's assets in compliance with prudential rules,

- Voluntary work means that the functions performed by the members of the governing body are free of charge,

- responsible participation requires the member to observe a certain loyalty to the institution and to other members21.

In Senegal, only 20% of the population, made up of the formal sector, is covered by a health insurance system, while the informal sector, which represents more than 80% of the population, is only covered to the extent of 7%28. The priority given to the financial accessibility of quality health services has been demonstrated by the governments that have succeeded one another in recent decades with the implementation of several programmes. This will has been materialized by the implementation of a National Health Development Plan (PNDS) 2009/2018, one of the strategic orientations of which is the reinforcement of the coverage of the health risk by emphasizing the vulnerable groups targeted to benefit from the Social Security Grant (BSF) and the Equal Opportunity Card (CEC), on the one hand, and the Emerging Senegal Plan (PSE), which serves as a reference framework for the State's action, on the other. Axis II of the PES, entitled *"Human capital, social protection and sustainable development",* aims to achieve a significant improvement in people's living conditions and a more sustained fight against social inequalities, while promoting the emergence of viable territories.15

In this context, the Universal Health Coverage (CMU) is an adaptation of the Senegalese government's CSU focused on the management of financial risk by orienting it towards the management of illness as a priority target. Senegal has adopted a CMU programme in line with the Government's desire to reduce inequalities in access to health care. Thus, the Ministry of Health and Social Action has developed a Strategic Plan for the Development of Health Coverage (PSD-CMU) 2013-2017 through an agency in charge of implementing the national CMU strategy, whose major orientations revolve around the development of MOHs, the reinforcement of free health care initiatives and collaboration with other sectors with a view to reforming health insurance institutions13[,15].

The Matam region currently has 26 health centres housed in its 26 communes, but the commitment of the local authorities is still lacking, even though health is a competence transferred to Senegal27. The majority of the health centres have no headquarters and the town halls do not necessarily support their development16. In addition, the precariousness of life and the particularly nomadic population make it difficult to implement the development strategy of the CSU through the health centres in this part of the country.

Through this study, we try to highlight the perceptions of the actors of the Matam MOH on the changes brought by this new policy of expansion of the MOH for the achievement of the UHC in Senegal.

Background to the study

It should be noted that low- and middle-income countries account for only 18% of global income and 11% of global health expenditure, but bear 93% of the world's burden of ill health. An effective and equitable health care system is an important instrument to break the vicious cycle of poverty and ill health. Sub-Saharan African countries have tried different ways of financing health care since independence18 . Catastrophic health expenditure is significantly associated with lack of health insurance and there is evidence that a massive expansion of health coverage can reduce catastrophic health expenditure among the population24.

According to the WHO, CHWs are a potential means to accelerate progress towards UHC3. Community-based health insurance systems through MOHs have experienced unprecedented growth in West and Central Africa since the 1990s. Several African countries have opted for the promotion of MI as a strategy to achieve UHC for the populations of the informal and rural sectors as well as the indigent populations28. Thus, we are increasingly witnessing a real progressive substitution of supply-based financing mechanisms by demand-side subsidy mechanisms. This reflects the will of African countries in general, and Senegal in particular, to make the MOH a strategic lever in the framework of poverty reduction and the extension of social and health protection3.

In Senegal, users pay for health care in two different ways, either by direct payment called Out-Of-Pocket Payment (OOP)[3] , or by contributing a portion of the cost supplemented by a system of financial protection ranging from the MS, Imputation Budgétaire (IB) for civil servants and state agents and their dependents, to the Institutions de Prévoyance Maladie (IPM), which is a supplementary insurance for salaried workers and their families, Retirement Provident Institutions (IPRES) for retirees in the formal sector up to free medical assistance for children under 5 years of age, people over 60 years of age, pregnant women with exempted caesarean section fees and kits, and certain chronic diseases requiring dialysis3.

As a reminder, the informal and rural sector, which represents more than 80% of the population, is covered by a health insurance system for only 7%. This is why the government has focused on this sector for the implementation of the CSU development strategy through the MS3.

Figure 1: Status of health coverage before 2013 in Senegal

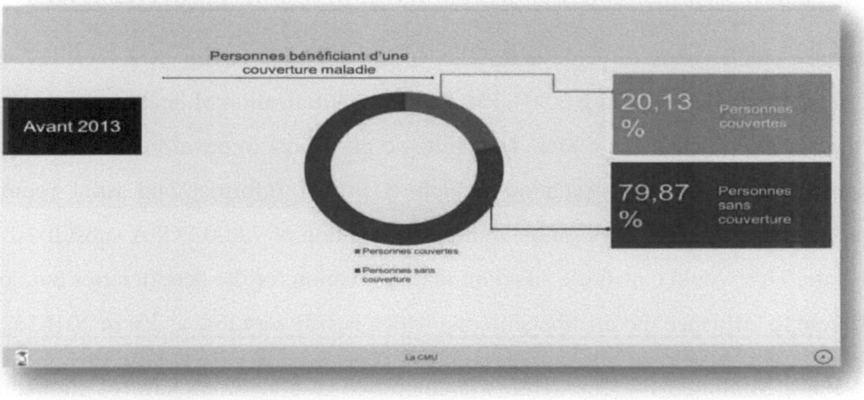

Source: Regional Agency of the CMU of Matam (2016)

Mutuals had existed in the past on the basis of solidarity and voluntary action at the community level. In the beginning, the term "*micro-health insurance*" was more widely used; it encompassed a wide variety of community-based systems aimed at the poor in the informal sector3,[16]. Among the micro-health insurance systems are the following:

- insurance provided by health care providers. A health centre or hospital may offer its potential users a membership fee that entitles them to either free or reduced prices for care. In most cases, members are not involved in the management of the system,

- insurance for non-profit medical transport. They are implemented, for example, by a municipality that has an ambulance. Each person who wants to benefit from the preferential rate has to contribute. The funds collected ensure that the cost of an emergency evacuation is free or reduced and are used to finance the operating costs of the vehicle,

- mutual health insurance. They combine the concepts of insurance, solidarity and participation3'[9]. The latter were targeted by the CMU in order to be revitalized.

Senegal's challenge is to achieve 75% coverage of basic health care by 2017, i.e. 11,442,260 people, including 6,804,331 with the revitalization of health care services as the second pillar of the CMU. The strategic plan aims to develop the MS for the remaining 80% of the population, which is in the informal and rural sectors. Beneficiaries contribute 50% of an annual contribution of 7,000 FCFA subsidized by the state. This would constitute an additional motivation for the beneficiaries but does not seem to influence the membership rate which is still very low at 3% in 201616.

The Basic Minimum Package (BMP) is composed of a basic package of care and a complementary package. The basic package includes services that are offered at the level of health posts and health centres. The complementary package includes services offered at the hospital level28 . It offers 80% coverage for consultations, analyses and hospital examinations, generic drugs and 50% for drugs supplied by private pharmacies19. According to the CMU regional office in Matam in 2013, as part of the implementation of the basic CMU through the MS, fourteen (14) pilot departments were selected at the rate of one department per region. Today, the CMU Agency is extending the approach to the remaining thirty-one (31) departments. A total of six hundred and seventy-one (671) MS have been set up with a total number of beneficiaries currently standing at 2,260,000 as at 31 December 2016, with 4,544,331 people still to be covered in order to reach the 2017 target19 described above.

In parallel with the establishment of the health centres and the targeted free health care, the government has set up a family security grant programme (BSF) aimed at beneficiaries of mutual insurance companies, with a subsidy of the total amount of the contribution and the co-payment for a total of 115,000 people19-20. Similarly, the granting of the Equal Opportunity Card (CEC) has made it possible to enrol disabled persons in the health insurance schemes, with the added advantage of a supplementary medical and equipment package.19

Study environment

The region of Matam is located in the north-east of Senegal, it covers an area of 29 616 km2. It is the second largest region in the country and is bordered to the north by the St Louis region, to the east by the Islamic Republic of Mauritania with which it shares the Senegal River, to the west by the Louga region and to the south by the Kaffrine and Tambacounda regions1[,15]. The relief is made up of plains and a few valleys with three agro-ecological zones: the "Dandé Mayo" (river valley), the "Ferlo" (lateritic zone) and the "Diéri" (sandy intermediate zone)[2,22]. The climate is dry and arid, with highs of more than 45°C during the first six months of the year. These conditions discourage agents from other parts of the country who are assigned to Matam, and they do not encourage the establishment of private structures such as clinics and pharmaceutical dispensaries. A second aspect reinforces this lack of interest in the region, namely its isolation and remoteness due to the distances involved and the defective or even absent road system. The economy of this region is essentially based on the agro-sylvopastoral field generating a trade centralized on the zone of Ourossogui without forgetting the important financial flow resulting from the transfers of capital of the emigrants. In 2013, it had about 58,462 households, 45.2% of which were living in poverty. The population is 630,703, which represents only 4.3% of the population of Senegal, with a sex ratio of 0.97. It is relatively young, 47.27% is under 15 years old, spread over three departments, five arrondissements and 26 communes with a density of 21 inhabitants per square kilometre2. At the beginning of last year, three pilot mutual insurance companies were launched, following the example of the entire country, and currently all the communes have their own MS1[,16]. The communal mutuals are grouped around departmental unions in each department. A regional union has been set up and the office has just been constituted during the organisation of the regional commission for monitoring the activities of the MS in the region which was held at the end of March 201716,[19]. However, this hierarchy does not allow for the transversal mutualisation of care, in other words, a member of a MOH cannot be cared for outside its agreed structures.

Existing financial protection plans

In the Matam region, there are four health coverage schemes, in line with national guidelines:

- Compulsory scheme for government employees, which includes (IB): Coverage of 80% of costs, excluding medicines, provided by approved health facilities.

- Compulsory scheme (IPM): Letter of guarantee, Coverage of benefits between 40 and 50%, Benefits provided mainly in private clinics and practices, Coverage of medicines in private pharmacies.

- Voluntary mutual insurance scheme (MS): Payment of the moderating ticket during the services, State subsidy around 50% for the classic membership and 100% for the BSF and CEC, Services made at the level of the agreed health structures.

- Medical assistance scheme (targeted free of charge): Identification and targeting of beneficiaries, free services at public health facilities, reimbursement of services by the State or technical and financial partners16,[19].

The regional CMU office is the body responsible for coordinating the activities of health-care providers and their buyers.

The health offer

Table 1: Staff ratios compared to health standards in 2016

RATIOS AND HEALTH STANDARDS

Human RMMIUI-<ES	Targets	Regional coverage	Gap	RUUroncu PNDS/OMS
26 Physicians	630 702 hts	1 doctor for 25,228 people	-38	1 doctor per 10,000 inhabitants (WHO)
2 gynaecologists	152 630 FAR	1 gynaecologist for 76 315 FAR		
0 pediatrician	249,379 children	0 pediatricians for 249,379 children		
86 Midwives	152 630 FAR	1 midwife for 1775 FAR	0	1 for 1500 TO 2000 FAR (PNDS)
3 chlrurgltiu tooth bed		1 dentist for 198,843 hts		
14S Inftnaten and nursing assistants	630702 b«	1 Nurse for 4350 hts	♦ 19	1 per 5000 hts (PNDS)
2 bvpitûut		1 hOpCul for 315,330 hu	.2	1 hospital per 150,000 inhabitants (WHO)
Health Centres		1 CS for 1S7 676 h"	0	1 CS per 100,000 to ISO,000 hrs" (NSDP)
90 health posts		1 PS for 7006 hts	- 36	1 SP per 5,000 hts (NSDP)

Source: Matam Medical Region (2017)

The Matam medical region manages four health districts. The department of Matam has two districts, while Kanel and Ranérou-Ferlo each have only one. The technical platform has been strengthened in recent years through development cooperation with the construction of several health posts and centres, especially in the Ferlo (Kanel and Ranerou). The staff has been strengthened to make up for this deficit, which is linked to the fact that health workers do not stay long because of the climatic difficulties described above, which makes the region one of the least attractive in the country.[8,16]

Organization of the Mutual Societies in the region

The MS in the region are created within the municipalities of the different departments. They are under the responsibility of local elected volunteers who hold the office of president. They are united at departmental level by a departmental union whose president is also democratically elected. The management bodies of both the MS and the departmental unions are the General Assembly (GA), which is held at least once a year, the Board of Directors, which determines the direction of the organisation and ensures that it is implemented, and a supervisory body made up of people elected by the GA. The Executive Board (EB) is chosen and is in charge of the daily management of the MS, it ensures the execution of the decisions of the GA. The EB is composed of the leaders including the president, the vice-president, the secretary and the treasurer who ensure the smooth running of the MS19.

Participating members of a health insurance scheme are natural persons or legal entities having subscribed to a group contract, who, in return for paying a contribution, are entitled to benefit from the social advantages and services offered by the health insurance scheme and to extend the right to their dependants. Fee-for-service payment is the one favoured by the Matam MOHs between 50% and 20% as a co-payment depending on the service21.

As a result, an agreement is signed with the health structures with the help of an agreement for the purchase of services. Depending on the level of care, the invoicing methods can go up to, at the level :

- of the health centres of : An amount per episode of illness, An amount per consultation, An amount per medical visit, A lump sum per member registered at the health centre, A budget.

- Hospitals: Fee-for-service or per service, Lump sum per day of hospitalization, Lump sum per duration of hospitalization.

Two payment methods combined, direct payment and third-party payment, keep the triangular relationship between the member, the provider and the MS21 in balance.

Figure 2: organization and functioning of the MS in the Matam region

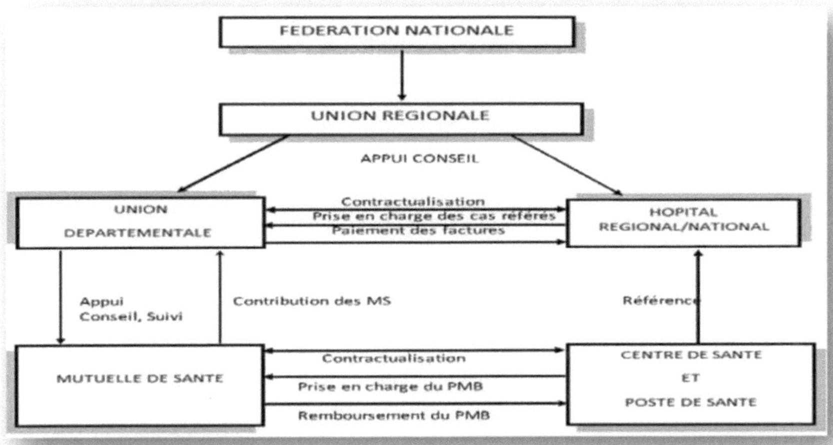

Source: regional office of the CMU of Matam (2017).

The new CMU guidelines in Senegal have been harmoniously oriented, beyond the reinforcement of compulsory insurance for formal people through the IB, the IPM and the IPRES, on two major axes, namely the targeted free health care policies and the revitalization of the MOHs, both of which are oriented towards informal and rural people28. Figure 2 shows the organization of the MOHs in the Matam region and their relationship with the health system to ensure better access for the population. Since independence, mutual insurance companies have existed, but not only were there not many of them throughout the country, but it was just the desire of a small part of the population to help each other, and they were not regulated. Nowadays, the new State guidelines harmonize, regulate and revitalize the MS. They aim at social equity, the whole population should have access to the quality care they need without being discriminated against, with a particular emphasis on solidarity and risk sharing28. However, in the implementation of this axis which concerns the MOHs, several equations remain to be solved in the sense that the start-up was done in a pilot phase with actors, elected community leaders who did not necessarily have experience in the sector and were often illiterate. The policies of revitalization and extension of the MOHs are not always internalized by the stakeholders and the coverage is theoretically pretentious, but in the application several obstacles are raised.

Figure 3: Conceptual model of health coverage through the MOHs in Matam

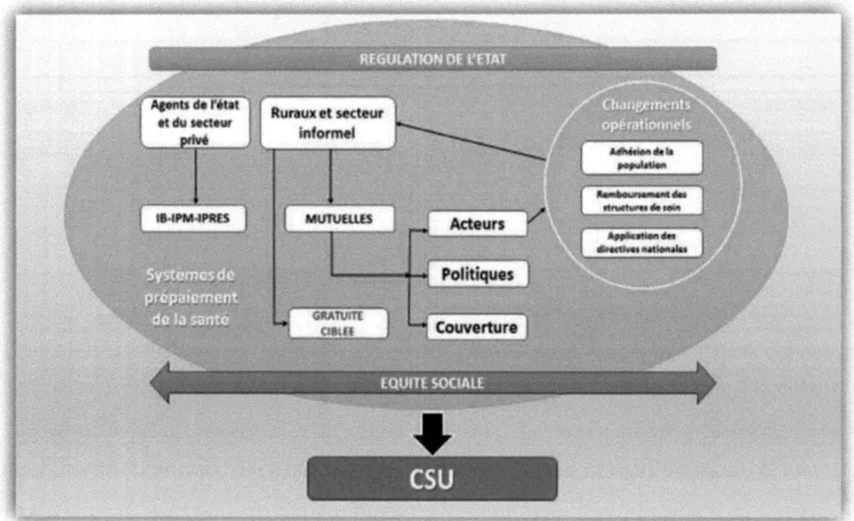

Source: the authors

The actors of the MOH, as responsible, must invest in all the operational changes brought by the new orientations of the state towards the CMU, namely :

- to encourage the population to join massively, a guarantee of the survival of the MS, in a context where the specificities of the region described above do not favour this enthusiasm necessary for its success.

- To manage the reimbursement of the structures that have signed up to the MS and to guarantee transparency in order to maintain this confidence, which is a sine qua non condition that determines the future of the MS.

- Apply and enforce the national guidelines on the establishment and management of a MS according to the state standards described above while being part of the network formed by the federated mutualist unions as defined in the PSD-CMU28.

The new orientations of the CMU leave gaps in its implementation at the operational level, in the daily experience of the actors of the MOH. These actors, made up of volunteers, often do not have proven experience in the management of MOHs and are often illiterate and are the linchpin of the development of the CMU through the MOHs.

Research Question

What are the changes expressed by the actors of the mutual health insurance schemes brought about by the implementation of the CMU in Matam?

Objectives of the study

This study mainly aims to explore the point of view of the actors on the development of the MOH in order to detect the organizational, technical and relational shortcomings and difficulties brought by the new orientations of the State in a context of expansion towards the CMU.

It will focus on aspects such as:

- The organizational character related to the daily management of the MS,
- ownership and implementation of national guidelines,
- the difficulties linked to the application of these new guidelines in the articulation between the MS, the structure under agreement and the member.
- The aspects of improving the daily life of the actors in the exercise of their function.

An analytical study was carried out among the staff of the MOHs, which made it possible to relate their daily professional experiences, practices and perceptions of the changes brought about by the implementation of the CSU with its national implementation standards. Indeed, it allowed to emphasize the discrepancies reported and which can constitute an added value to the evolution towards the CSU and allow to have a glimpse on its future.

Methodology of the study

This is a qualitative study that explored the perceptions of mutual health insurance stakeholders in the Matam region on the changes brought about by the implementation of the CSU.

An exploratory phase was preceded by guided interviews with :

- The Director of Health Insurance in Dakar, who told us that a preliminary study had been conducted on the feasibility of expanding the health insurance scheme as part of the universal health insurance scheme. This study, based on a survey of households, had made it possible to set the amount of contributions deemed sustainable and to determine the share of state subsidy, which is currently 50% of the contribution and 100% for the vulnerable groups described above.

- The Regional Chief Medical Officer because he represents the regional health authority and can provide us with strategic guidance and useful data for our investigation. The medical region ensures the transmission of data to the national level as it is the strategic body of the region in terms of health. It ensures close collaboration with the regional office of the CMU and with the help of local partners, it allows the monitoring of the activities of the MOHs and facilitates their collaboration with the points of service provision (PPS) of the region.

- The Director of the Regional Office of the CMU for a theoretical deepening and a better orientation on the axes and processes of development of the MOH. This meeting brought out the newly defined major orientations of the CMU, namely the new initiative of free health care and the expansion of the MOH. The start of the demonstration phase of the "*Decentralization and Health Insurance*" project through the development of the MOHs (14 pilot departments, one department per region). Major innovations are introduced (State subsidies, extension of the care package, strengthening of regulations)[13]. The challenge is major, given that most of the actors are volunteers and sometimes have management difficulties due to illiteracy. The monthly payment of reimbursements should reduce the delays in the economic management of mutual insurance companies through their federation at the departmental level. Alternatives such as the State paying the salaries of a manager for each health insurance fund and two administrators at the departmental union level are new ways established by the State to facilitate the development of health insurance funds. This came out of the last regional monitoring committee of the MOHs organised in Matam at the end of March, in which we took part.

- The Regional Focal Point of the CMU in Matam for a more operational vision of the implementation of the CSU and a better targeting of our survey population. This resulted in a clarification of the new orientations, namely the harmonization of the MS, the organization of the executive offices and the enrolment of vulnerable groups (BSF and CEC).

Sampling

In-depth semi-directive interviews were carried out with the actors of the health insurance schemes in the three departments of the region in order to ensure the diversity and heterogeneity of the sample. One or two people were selected in a reasoned way per mutual until saturation.

Method of data collection

Visits to the three departments were made by making an appointment with the presidents of the MOHs to conduct these individual interviews. Out of a total of 26 MOHs, distributed as follows: 10 MS in the department of Matam, 12 MS in the department of Kanel and 4 MS in the department of Ranerou, we reached saturation with 18 interviews. Two interviews were eliminated because of problems in using the information, since after the translation into French of the content initially in Poulhar, the information was biased in our opinion and therefore eliminated for reasons of accuracy. Two MS presidents refused to participate in the interview, claiming that they did not want to affirm anything because they were only at the beginning of their work. We ended up with a participation rate of 70% and an acceptance rate of 89% for all the MS in the region. The following topics were discussed using an interview guide (see

Appendix 1)

- difficulties related to membership (traditional and vulnerable groups),
- the realities around coordination between structures and members,
- the completeness and attractiveness of the MS coverage,
- the conditions for carrying out the tasks assigned, reflecting their motivation to support the MS expansion project.

The data collected was processed and analysed using encoding techniques with inductive codes on the content of the collected speeches7 . Indeed, all the interviews were first transcribed and entered into the computer. A first reading allowed us to identify the relevant themes and a tree structure was thus developed (Figure 4).

Results

The interviews lasted between half an hour and three quarters of an hour and the predominant discourse revolved around the management and the weight of responsibility of the actors within the MS. the content analysis brought out several themes, the most important of which are: commitment to the MS, the training of the actors, the state subsidy, confidence in the MS, the overload of work with the voluntary work and the benefit conferred by the MS.

Table 2 summarizes the attributes identified by the stakeholders on the changes brought about by the expansion of the health services through the CMU in Matam.

A large number of actors reported a strong commitment to the development of their MOH. In fact, most of them expressed their dedication since the revitalization of the MOH. According to one manager: "*Apart from my job, I am dedicated to the mutual health insurance scheme*", another said: "*First of all, I was the initiative chairman from the start and I am committed. In my mutual, I play the role of president and manager at the same time*.

Figure 4: Matrix of the perceptions of stakeholders in Matam on operational changes in relation to the MS in Matam.

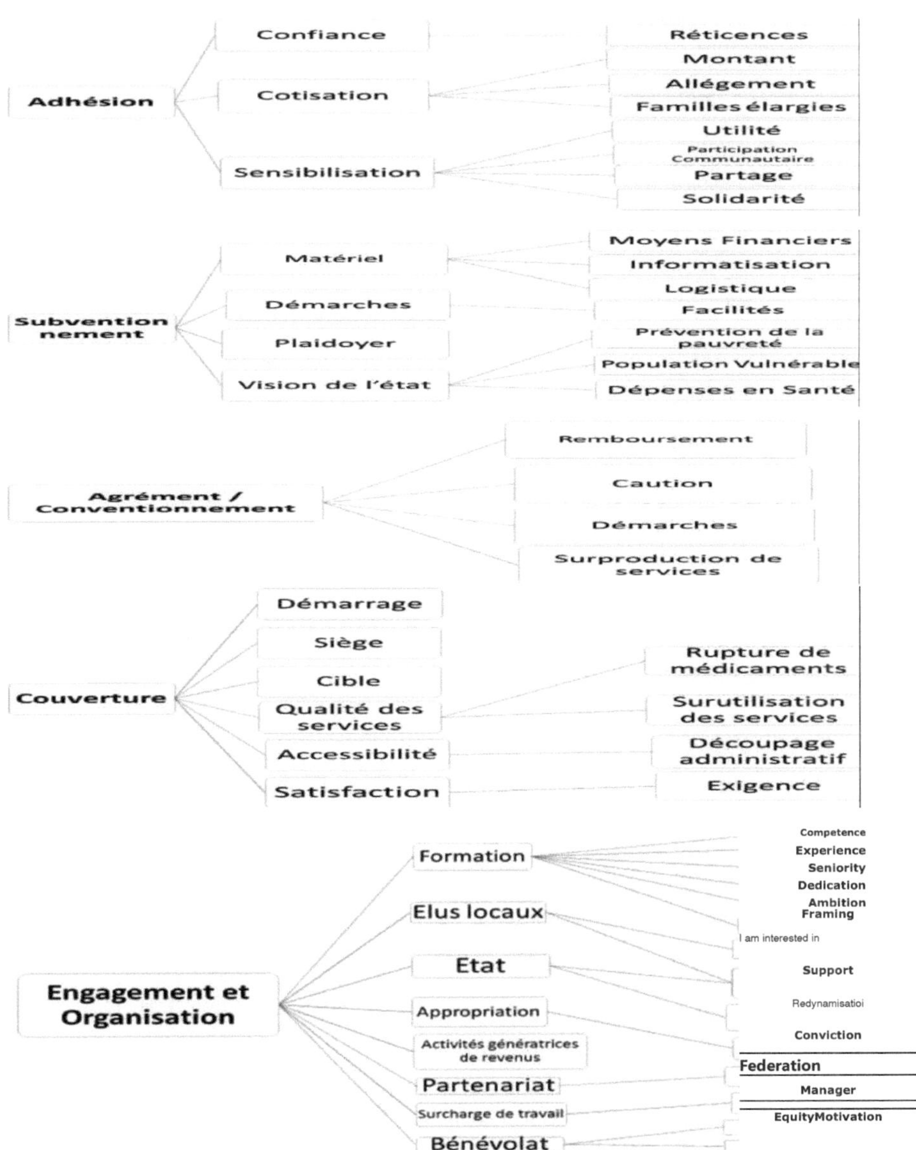

Source: the authors

Moreover, the commitment of the state was reported by several MS leaders. Indeed, according to one president: "*All these current orientations that did not exist before are an excellent thing and prove the government's commitment to change things*", according to another: "It is *difficult to get health care anywhere in the world. The fact that the state is committed to helping the most vulnerable populations to have health care is to be welcomed.* However, the actors do not feel this commitment at the level of the MS on the part of the local elected officials. Indeed, one president exclaimed: "What is missing is the commitment of local elected officials", according to another president: "*Local actors must be more committed (the departmental council, local authorities, etc.)*". However, this impression is not totally shared because some of them explained that some town halls have made efforts to support their MS. In fact, according to a president who is also a municipal delegate: "*We have just voted a budget for our MOH because health is of primary interest to us because health has been transferred, so we are interested in anything that can alleviate the suffering of the population. We really need much more commitment to the MOHs because the vision is good, the content is good, but much more support is needed*", an official said in this sense: "*We had received 500,000F from the mayor in terms of subsidy but it is not enough to start*".

Moreover, this commitment of the actors is limited by the inadequacy of training, which they unanimously pointed out. Many of them deplored the lack of updating since the initial training sessions with the Mutual Initiative Committees (MICs), which were set up at the local community level, as an initiation to the launching of the MS. The presidents, elected by the people, were trained on the basic concepts of mutuality, the process of setting up and the fundamental parameters. The members of the elected bodies were then trained in administrative and financial management. It is in this sense that one MS president exclaimed: "What is *missing is the training of elected representatives. Since the IMCs, there has been practically no training. Capacity building is a problem*", another spoke in the same vein: "*Since the initial training sessions, which were quick, there has been no updating or refresher courses. So there are problems at this level.* For some presidents, this problem can even compromise the work in the MS. One of them exclaims: "*What makes the task difficult is the lack of training of the members who make up the office of the MOH, we have a treasurer who does not have the capacity for financial management and accounting. We have a treasurer who doesn't have the financial management and accounting skills, and that's a problem. Without training it is not possible*. Consequently, many recommendations targeted this lack of training, in fact, according to one official: "*Training would be welcome to strengthen capacities. We have a manager who is there but is not trained*", another confirmed: "*The capacities of mutual agents should be strengthened in terms of training. Without computer skills, it is difficult to manage the tools of the Ms*".

Moreover, despite the commitment of the state and the initial training, the actors of the MS unanimously complained about the delay of the subsidy. Many presidents saw this delay as a factor blocking the start of the MOHs. In this sense, one president stated: "*We cannot start without the subsidies because if people go for treatment at the PPS level and we cannot reimburse them, it creates a blockage. So we need the state to pay the subsidies, we can start and the memberships will follow*", followed by another: "*The subsidies are not yet available and these delays are also handicapping us*", a vice-president of a health ministry confirmed: "*The major difficulties are linked to the delay in subsidies, the lack of training and the lack of awareness*", another said: "*The state subsidises but not in time, there are many delays and this does not allow us to take care of the members properly*". Some even reported an accumulation of this delay from year to year. Indeed, according to an official in charge of the management of a MS: "*The slowness is rather at the level of the state which is slow to send the subsidies, we did not receive 2016 even less 2017 at this moment and this limits us in our prerogatives*". According to other actors, this is a way of putting them at odds with the population because the state asks them to enrol the identified vulnerable populations (BSF and CEC) without their subsidy being paid to the MOH. One chairman said: "*We have started to enrol TSOs and CECs and there is enthusiasm, but the subsidies should not be long in coming, otherwise it is a risk. The people know that the lists of TSOs and CECs are with us. This puts us in trouble with the people*. It is in this sense that the actors recommended that the state should do everything to be up to date with the subsidies. Indeed, a president suggested: "*What is urgent to do is to send the subsidies on time*". Insisting on the promptness of the grant, a chairman said: "*The state must be prompt in the grants so as not to drown this momentum*" and addressing the same issue another official supported: "*The promptness of the grant would be essential because we only received an initial grant to make the photos and maps for the TSOs and CECs. If they paid the grant money very soon, we would have a fairly solid and secure start-up fund that would allow us to get off to a good start, but this is not the case*. However, some actors attributed these delays to management difficulties and the transmission of accounting documents, invoices and reports. In fact, according to one president: "*To reduce the delays in the state subsidy, we need to do the job properly. These delays are partly due to us because all the documents are not forwarded on time and this is still the problem of management. We don't have a manager and we don't have the capacity to do the job properly*.

In any case, these difficulties give rise to problems mentioned by the stakeholders that are linked to trust. With regard to users, they explained that trust was initially demonstrated during the election of members of the MOH management bodies. According to one chairman: "*The chairmen of the MOHs are elected by the population based on their trust*", another spoke in the same vein: "*I am responsible, it is the people who elected me*". And they are aware of this, as one leader attested: "*My greatest concern is that the project succeeds because I have the trust of those who chose me*. However, with regard to structures such as the MS, it is more a question of a lack of confidence generated by the accumulation of previous unsuccessful experiences, as one actor stated: "*People used to contribute to other things that did not succeed and now they no longer have confidence*". According to the actors, it is rather caution or mistrust that generates a certain reluctance to join the MS. According to one of the presidents: "It's *like when I spoke at the last meeting on the MOH, I said that there were facilities but the populations are still reluctant to the idea of the MOH*", another MOH president insisted: "*The main difficulty is trust. Among us Soninke (the dominant ethnic group in the Senegal River Valley), people only come in if they see results. They have to see the first ones doing well first before they put their hands in*. Thus, the lack of trust is seen by the actors as a block to the expansion of the MOHs because it decreases adherence, which decreases the health coverage of the population. In this sense, another president said: "*It is a blockage because people want to contribute but they do not have confidence and we want the population to be covered*. This lack of confidence would also influence the low level of contributions and slow down contracting. According to one president: "*This means that the population does not have complete confidence in the system and this is reflected in membership and the renewal of contributions*". This was echoed by a departmental union president who said: "*I insisted a lot during the meeting on facilitating the signing of agreements because they help to build confidence in the population and boost membership and membership renewal*. However, strategies have been developed by actors to fight against this lack of confidence, namely awareness-raising, as stated by a leader of a MOH: "*The most important point is to make them see that the money is not managed by the state but rather by their own sons in the village and that for any contribution, the state has given the same amount as*

That was our solution to increase people's confidence so that they would adhere a little more and that had an effect. That was our solution to increase people's confidence so that they would adhere a little more and that had an effect", another, from a commercial point of view, proposed: "*We can also organise activities that generate resources to make the MS profitable, it's a question of marketing too. You have to know how to sell your product, that's what makes the MS attractive. We think we can build loyalty among our members because we will generate enough trust for the population to find their way around*. In general, the stakeholders see a bright future for the MS if they manage to gain the trust of the population. According to one stakeholder: "*The MOHs have a future if the start-up is well done, it would give confidence to the populations in order to increase membership*". Moreover, this lack of confidence is also manifested to different degrees with regard to service delivery structures such as hospitals and private pharmacies, according to the opinions of the actors. In fact, in hospitals, a deposit of a mutually defined amount is required as a guarantee and working capital, which is renewed each time the alert threshold is reached. According to a president of a departmental union: "*We have paid a deposit at the health centre level*", and another one: "*And moreover, it is planned to deposit money in the form of a deposit at the level of the service structures to avoid these problems of reimbursement among others*". Concerning private pharmacies, the lack of confidence was expressed in the content of the agreement contracts according to the actors. A manager of the MS exclaimed: "*The conventions have not yet been signed because there has been reluctance, especially on the part of pharmacists who do not have confidence in the content of the convention.*

In parallel to this confidence, the actors unanimously reported the work overload. Indeed, they expressed the enormous volume of work involved in managing a MS. According to one president: "There are *many tools and all of them must be kept up to date and it is a huge job*". For some, it means that they have to perform several functions in the mutual society and even beyond, as one actor said: "*I am the treasurer, I manage the mutual society's funds, and at the regional level, I am an advisor to the mutual societies in the department and I provide technical support to the other mutual societies. I also do training, capacity building and advocacy at the level of the authorities and partners*", according to another: "*In my mutual, I play the role of president and manager at the same time*" and another official replies: "*To do the work, we are obliged to run here and there to keep the registers up to date. The staff under our responsibility are getting more and more tired and we can't keep them.* The absence of a manager in the MOHs makes the chairpersons responsible and they end up taking over from him. According to their accounts, a manager's salary is not provided for anywhere and they do not work for free, even though managing money when you are not paid can constitute a risk (misappropriation of funds, risk of being assaulted, loss of money, etc.). In this sense, one president said: "*When you don't have enough funds, it is always difficult, especially when you have a president who is a volunteer and a manager without a salary with a mutual that does not have enough resources and wants to develop.* Another said: "*Imagine a manager who is not well paid and who manages the population's money, you can imagine all that can happen... ah, I'll let you imagine it yourself in this context of poverty*. Moreover, many of them demanded that a manager be indispensable, according to one actor: "*We don't have a manager and we don't have the capacity to do the job properly, otherwise we won't make it.* Based on these observations, most of the stakeholders recommended that a manager be recruited for each health ministry, because, according to one official, "*a manager must be hired permanently and paid by the state or by the mutualists*. In addition, this work overload is manifested in the very archaic way in which the health offices are managed. The actors unanimously decried the replacement of the numerous registers with more adequate computer equipment, in addition to the lack of headquarters for a good number of them. According to one official: "*We lack a place to work, the headquarters is missing. We can't work without a seat. The other problem is the equipment which is archaic. We need more modern means because the sheets are a crazy job and they can be destroyed*. Moreover, the work is not uniformly distributed and depends on the skills of the members of the office at the level of the MS. In this sense, one official said: "*There is a problem with the office, which is made up of 12 members, and only three of them are active in the management of the MS*. However, this multiplicity of things to do raised the issue of volunteering, which was unanimously considered to be related to the work overload and not in line with the current situation of the MS. In this vein, one president recalled: "*We could just add our desire for mutuals to develop in Matam and changing the volunteer system would be a key element in the development of mutuals*", while another added: "*Volunteering is not sustainable because everything depends on me and I cannot take care of my entire team of 7 people during meetings. There are a lot of meetings and there is always more work to do than travel. Really, it won't work with volunteers*. Moreover, the actors see it as a threat to the expansion of the MS in the long run. According to one president: "*We came in as volunteers, but it can't continue. We have to be motivated, housed, have logistical means and above all paid. Volunteering will not continue, people will refuse in the long run*", another confirmed: "*The question of volunteering handicaps us, the majority of the actors risk abandoning the MS because at present we sacrifice our professional life for the MS, leaving our resources behind and what do we gain*? Before the CMU, the people in charge of the mutuals were mostly volunteers, and some actors think that returning to this form of responsibility would be the beginning of a solution. On this basis, a regional union president stated: *"Moving towards voluntary work would be a first step towards motivation, but people could quickly become discouraged and it would not be beneficial for the mutuals"*.

In short, the new orientations of the MOH are perceived as favourable to the improvement of the health of the populations while protecting them from poverty according to the great majority of the actors. According to a manager: "*All these changes have an impact on our work in the sense that we now have axes to exploit for the benefit of the populations and this is beneficial. People need it*", according to another official: "*These new orientations are positively perceived*". In addition, they gave a certain advantage to the MS actors in their work. Indeed, one official stated: "*The procedures have been facilitated in the conventions with the health post and the Matam health centre and the people who have benefited from care motivate other people to come and register and join*", according to another: "*These new orientations really facilitate our work in the health centres*". Some workers even spoke of a revolution in their lives and work. Indeed, one leader said, "*These changes have revolutionized our lives and our work. Imagine all the things that the state is taking over and given the importance of the act, it's all new and it's really important.* In addition, they also confer an advantage on the population, a large proportion of the respondents considered that joining a health insurance scheme is favourable to the family's economy and improves health. According to one actor: "That is *to say that it already allows the population to save money, that is already good. Then for the women who did not have the possibility to have check-ups and ultrasounds. They used to pay 10,000 francs for each of these examinations, now they pay 2,000 francs, do you see what this does? It allows them to save money and to live their lives peacefully. They are not afraid to go to the hospital now. It's also a motivating factor and it allows for better health. I find these new orientations positive because if everything is well structured, it would allow a better adhesion*". These guidelines mainly target the rural and informal sector populations and it is in this sense that an official confirmed: "In *relation to the CMU, these guidelines have come to help the weakest populations, those with low incomes, since the president came up with this idea, there has been an improvement in health. Before, it was only the formal sector that was taken care of, now the informal and rural sectors are interested.* Moreover, they help to fight against social inequity and access to health care for the population, as one official underlined: "*It's a way of taking care of people from different social levels. All people are equal in this country and it was time to think about the most vulnerable, it is really an opportunity to seize. People who want health care and not money now have a chance like everyone else. And all this without having to resort to debt or sell their luggage*. Moreover, the changes have created a general excitement and interest among the population, a president confirmed: "There have *been very important changes in the MS. Before, they were not as dynamic and now everyone is talking about them, but the problem of funding remains*. The actors also perceived a general interest in these orientations. According to one MOH president: "*Before, they were civil servants' mutual insurance companies, now it is the government's will and the support of the president of the republic to really move towards CMU, we are moving towards the generalization of MOHs throughout Senegal and it is the government's will*", according to a more global vision of an actor: "*I find them very good, they are good acts and good reflections, without health we cannot develop. The President of the Republic wants to have more than 75% of the population covered by 2017*", another actor replied: "*The meetings organised allow us to standardise our work and share our experience. Centralization at the regional level is a strong point. Organizing around the departmental union and soon the regional union is like a federation of mutuals.*

Table 2: Identified themes expressed by stakeholders in Matam on operational changes in relation to the MOH.

Themes	Situations prior to the implementation of the CMU	Current situations
1. the in Commitment to the MS	A. Organized leaders B. Lack of commitment from the state C. Lack of involvement of local elected officials D. Very few mutuals with different functions	A. Dedication of the actors B. Commitment of the state - Revitalization - Standardization - Regulation - Prioritization C. Weak involvement of local elected officials D. Existence of a MS in each commune
2. Training of actors	A. No standardized training B .... C. Managers hired	A. Initial training - Basic concepts - Implementation process - Basic parameters - Administrative and financial management B. Lack of updating or continuing education C. Untrained managers
3. The state subsidy	A. No subsidy B. No accounting document to be transmitted to the state	A. Delays in the payment of the grant B. Difficulties in the management and transmission of accounting documents
4. Trust in the MS	A. Members chosen at the will of someone or a group of people B. Reasoned and convenient choice of members and structures C. Independent Alternatives	A. Members of the management bodies elected by the community B. Mistrust or caution with regard to the MS of users to join and structures to agree C. State-regulated alternatives
5. Work overload and volunteering	A. Appointed officialsand everyone has their role B. Internal management C. Existence of a seat D. Volunteering is not a basic principle E.............	A. Cumulation of volunteer leaders' duties B. Standardized management tools C. Not often a seat D. Management based on the principle of volunteerism E. Inadequacy of volunteering
6. The advance of mutuality	A. More convenience in health care B. No standardization	A. Poverty prevention B. Standardization facilitates the work of the actors
	C. Oriented towards formal agents and some local initiatives	C. Rural and informal oriented

Source: the authors

Discussions and recommendations

Our study aimed mainly to explore the stakeholders' point of view on the development of the MHOs in order to identify the organizational, technical and relational shortcomings and difficulties brought about by the State's new orientations in a context of expansion towards the CMU. It attempted to answer the question: "What changes were expressed by mutual health insurance stakeholders as a result of the implementation of CMU in Matam? The exploitation of the results oriented us mainly towards the following themes.

Revitalization of the MS

The revitalisation of the MOH has given rise to a very strong commitment on the part of the actors who have taken ownership of the management since their election. It is found in the literature that individuals who feel an affective commitment develop a very positive attitude towards the organisation, reflected in a desire to contribute spontaneously to its good functioning30 . This was reflected in a shared feeling on the part of the actors to make the MS work despite the difficult conditions in the region. The fact that they are elected by the communities reinforces this feeling of responsibility among the stakeholders, which even pushes them to use their own funds to develop the MS. This commitment is also noted on the part of the state, which is reflected in all the new guidelines that regulate the health centres with the aim of achieving universal coverage of the population. The state has set itself the objective of extending health coverage to 75% of the population employed in the informal and rural sectors by 2017 in the PSD-CMU. The concrete translation of this objective calls for the involvement of each actor who must do everything possible to ensure effective and efficient coverage for the target populations28. However, there is a large gap between the state's expectations regarding the involvement of local authorities in the expansion of the MOH and their actual level of commitment. Indeed, local authorities host the MOHs in a context where health is a decentralized competence27 and they are expected to support a departmental health solidarity fund jointly with the State and available in each department to support the expansion of the PMBs and the care of indigent and vulnerable groups28 , which has not been achieved. This factor could slow down the development of MOHs in Matam. This situation was encountered in Rwanda where local authorities and opinion leaders were little involved in the process of setting up mutual insurance companies and awareness was insufficient25. In the logic of action of the PSD- CMU, it is planned to advocate with local authorities for the care of the indigent and vulnerable groups through the MS28 , which could be the beginning of a solution.

The grant

Our study identified the delay in the state subsidy as a hindrance to the start-up and proper functioning of the MS. In fact, the actors claimed not to have received payment for the years 2016 and 2017. This situation raises a big question mark because in fact, the share that the state covers, 50% of the classic contributions and 100% for vulnerable people (BSF and CEC), is substantial. Between 2013 and 2017, the state, together with local authorities and Technical Financial Partners, invested an average of 80,685 million CFA francs28 , of which we have not found details of the pooling (allocation of resources), which raises the question of the transparency of health financing, on the one hand, and on the other hand, contradicts the statements made by the actors about the lack of involvement of local authorities mentioned above. At the time of its elaboration, the PSD-CMU had foreseen that the Departmental Solidarity Funds (DSFs) would fulfill three functions such as a partial subsidy to extend benefit packages and to promote the pooling of large risks of community MOHs at the departmental level; targeted subsidies to ensure the care of indigent and vulnerable groups through community MOHs; and guarantee mechanisms to promote group membership through partnerships between community MOHs and decentralized financing institutions (microfinance, microcredit, and savings).[28] In addition, our study showed that the procedures for receiving this state subsidy are too cumbersome, in terms of bureaucracy and transmission of reports and invoices, and even for the enrolment of vulnerable people, which may explain the delay in the collection of the MOHs. The latter do not get off the ground because of the lack of funds to ensure their activities. Furthermore, the allocation of a headquarters and the computerisation of the management of the MOHs would be a feasible alternative, and is even decried by the actors, which would save time and quality in the procedures for reimbursement and subsidies.

Membership and agreement

The low level of adherence to the MOH in Matam can be explained, among other things, by the population's lack of confidence in the management of the MOH. In addition, it was found that in the "Soninké" environment, the dominant ethnic group in the Senegal River valley, people adhere when they see that others have already done so and that they are satisfied. The literature has revealed that people frequently adopt a cautious attitude when launching a SM, preferring to observe before adhering12. Awareness raising in terms of trust would help to make the population aware and to fight against these reluctances by insisting on the values that once founded our communities such as solidarity and sharing through CP in order to internalize the usefulness of the MOH in the management of health risks, especially when we know that joining a MOH has a positive effect on the individual's health status. Thus, joining a health insurance scheme increases the probability that the individual's health status will be better by about 9% compared to those who do not join15. Moreover, the massive adhesion and the principles of solidarity and mutual aid which characterize African communities are limited by financial constraints26. Thus, the introduction of a differentiated contribution modality between the richest and the least rich would make it possible to reinforce this confidence and the principle of vertical and horizontal equity in the financing of the health insurance schemes as well as the principle of solidarity which constitutes the basis of the mutualist movement3. Moreover, the perspective of compulsory contributions could be envisaged through the new information and communication technologies. In fact, we found that almost everyone in Senegal has a mobile phone that is constantly powered and that even offers a multitude of commercial functions, including a contribution to a mutual health insurance plan, following the example of Gabon, which has instituted a 10% levy on mobile phones29. However, our study revealed that the means and the geographical context do not facilitate this awareness. The state would benefit from using the media to reach the maximum number of people, especially in less accessible areas, and to interest telephone companies in a partnership that would be beneficial and profitable for all. Similarly, the lack of confidence of the structures towards the MOH and the various experiences in the reimbursement have obliged the managers of the health structures to ask for a deposit from the managers of the MOH which would serve as a working capital and a guarantee at the same time. This situation is a handicap insofar as the funds are not always available in the health centres. The private structures are more suspicious, according to the head of the association of pharmacists in Kanel, who stated on their behalf at the last meeting of the monitoring committee of the MOHs in which we took part, the contracts were not clear and did not suit them, which is why they did not sign them. Moreover, inconsistencies were noted in the agreement because the study showed that the lack of portability and transversality for members, particularly nomads in the region, did not allow them to be taken in charge in the reception areas where the structures were not in agreement with their MOH, which strongly contributed to the low membership. However, it is planned that a framework agreement be signed between the departmental union of mutual health insurance and each of the health districts to harmonize the contractual arrangements between the community mutual health insurance and the health posts and health centers of the district, and the provisions concerning mandatory referral and portability of coverage within the department28 , which is not effective according to the respondents.

Work overload

The work overload would discourage the leaders of the MS, whose volunteer status no longer corresponds to current requirements. The accumulation of functions would be at the root of this work overload in the MS. Indeed, the presidents are elected through the manifest trust of the populations and this increases the degree of responsibility at their level. The lack of staff capacity, in this case the absence of a manager and the lack of work organisation (job description and tasks) would be a factor aggravating the situation. The lack of training would be a handicap because the managers, even if they are willing to do everything, have neither the necessary skills to do the work on a daily basis, nor to transfer these skills to a subordinate actor who would be willing to support the management of the MS. It is found in the literature that an individual's confidence in his or her ability to learn and develop skills is significantly associated with his or her perceptions of the intrinsic and extrinsic instrumentality of training and the valence of improving his or her leadership style31. Thus, good leadership training would contribute to the development of the MS. In addition, many chairpersons of the MOHs have decried the lack of financial motivation and even the use of own funds to manage the MOHs, most of whom see no future if this orientation is not reviewed. According to some authors, the challenges faced by community MOHs in Senegal include the lack of subsidized salaries for the staff of mutuals, the development of governance structures through mutualist federations, ensuring that MOHs resonate with the values of community solidarity, and greater transparency in national policies.17 Transforming community management of MOHs into a "*community enterprise*" orientation in which everyone is a shareholder would increase involvement and hence ownership by the people. In addition, decision-makers should support the recruitment and capacity building of one manager per MOH. As health is a competence transferred to Senegal, local authorities should be more involved in the development of the MOHs27.

The benefits of MS

Stakeholders reported that joining a MOH conferred enormous benefits on its members. The MOH improves the health of the population while protecting them from impoverishment by health expenses15. The new guidelines have facilitated the work of the actors in the harmonized approaches and shared experiences within the departmental and regional unions28. In addition, the protection targets informal, rural and vulnerable populations, which means that the MOHs are fighting against social inequalities in health by allowing access to quality care for the most disadvantaged.

Limits

Our study was severely limited in execution by the lack of time and human, material and financial resources. The lack of relevant literature is a recurrent problem in our countries which limits our exploration and hinders us in the scientific evidence.

Conclusions

Taking into account the perceptions of stakeholders is a key issue in the development of MOHs to achieve UHC in Senegal and particularly in Matam. The initial objective was to collect the views of the stakeholders on the changes brought about by the new policy for revitalizing the MOHs. Our work allowed us to detect discrepancies between the expectations of the national directives and the daily experience of the actors. Support for the MOHs is severely limited by the population's lack of confidence. This is aggravated by the lack of training and motivation of the actors who, for most of the respondents, find voluntary work unsuitable and unsustainable. As the state subsidies only arrive very late, the repercussions are felt, among other things, in the agreements, which further widen the gap of restraint and scepticism of the population towards the MOH. All these elements contribute to weakening this system, which is still in its infancy. The decision-makers would gain by finding a new form of participatory but motivating management of the MOHs by the community actors by involving the local authorities in taking charge of those responsible. Several alternatives can be envisaged, ranging from the transformation of the MS into a "community enterprise" where everyone would be a shareholder, to the involvement of telecommunication companies by making membership mandatory through reassuring legislation.

Bibliography

1. Report of the National Agency of Statistics and Demography. Report Matam Region. 2013. [Internet]. [cited 30 Dec 2016]. Available from: http://www.ansd.sn/index.php?option=com regions&view=region&layout=indicators&id=12#.

2. Report of the Regional Service of Statistics and Demography of Matam. REGIONAL ECONOMIC AND SOCIAL SITUATION. 2013. [Internet]. [cited 30 Dec 2016]. Available from: http://www.ansd.sn/ressources/ses/SES-Matam-2013.pdf.

3. Sagna O, Seck I, Dia AT, Sall FL, Diouf S, Mendy J, et al. Study of user preference on strategies for developing universal health coverage through mutual health insurance in the Ziguinchor region of southwest Senegal. Bulletin of the Society of Exotic Pathology. august 2016;109(3):195,206.

4. WHO 58th World Health Assembly adopts resolution on cancer prevention and control. [Internet]. WHO. [cited 30 Dec 2016]. Available from : http://www.who.int/mediacentre/news/releases/2005/pr wha05/en/.

5. Bamako Initiative Review. World Bank. 2016. [Internet]. [cited 30 Dec 2016]. Available from : http://documents.worldbank.org/curated/en/417091468763473890/pdf/303780HNP0BamakoInitiativeReview.pdf.

6. WHO | What is universal coverage? World Health Organization Report. 2016. [Internet]. WHO. [cited 13 Nov. 2016]. Available from: http://www.who.int/health financing/universal coverage definition/en/.

7. Methods of analysis and interpretation of qualitative research: state of the art in marketing (PDF Download Available) [Internet]. [cited 29 Jan 2017].

Available on : https://www.researchgate.net/publication/238711815 methods of analysis and interpretation of qualitative studies state of the art in marketing

8. Tapsirou Hamath BA - Geography of the health care system in the region of Matam in Senegal: what adequacy between the supply and demand of care - [Internet]. Memoire Online. [cited 13 Jan 2017]. Available from: http://www.memoireonline.com/11/12/6496/m Geographie-du-systeme-de-soins-dans-la-region-de-Matam-au-Senegal-quelle-adequation-entre-l-o6.html

9. Waelkens - Health-mutuals-in-Africa-sub-saharan-state Places-and-think-about-a-research-agenda.pdf [Internet]. [cited 2017 Mar 5]. Available from : https://www.researchgate.net/profile/Bart Criel/publication/27597585 Mutual health care in sub-Saharan Africa Saharan State of play and reflections on a research agenda/links/09e4150c0d4d350453000000/Les-mutuelles-de-sante-en-Afrique-sub-saharienne-Etat-des-lieux-et-reflexions-sur-un-agenda-de-recherche.pdf

10. Mutual health insurance in Africa and quality of care in services: a dynamic interaction (PDF Download Available) [Internet]. ResearchGate. [cited 5Apr2017]. Available from : https://www.researchgate.net/publication/27597475 Mutual health insurance in Africa and quality of care in the services a dynamic interaction.

11. Advocating for universal health coverage, UHC_FRvs1. 2013. [Internet]. [cited 13 Nov 2016]. Available from: http://www.who.int/health financing/UHC FRvs1.pdf?ua=1

12. Determinants of membership in mutual health insurance in Africa Sub-Saharan Africa: an inventory of empirical work - Cairn.info [Internet]. [cited 20March2017]. Available from: http://www.cairn.info.ezproxv.ulb.ac.be/article.php7ID ARTICLE=MED 153 0007

13. S.B. Badiane. Universal Health Coverage in Senegal: Status of implementation and prospects. Society of Exotic Pathology; 2013. [Internet] Available from: https://

spe-smanlf-2013 .sciencesconf.org/27993

14. World Health Report 2013: Research for Coverage
universal health. World Health Organization, Geneva 2013 [Internet]. [cited 22 March 2017]. Available from: http://apps.who.int/medicinedocs/documents/s22233fr/s22233fr.pdf

15. Ndongo JCA, Mahieu P-A, Nanfosso RT. Mutual health insurance and health status of populations in Cameroon: a survey conducted in the Central Region to estimate the effect of membership in a mutual health insurance scheme on self-reported health status. Journal of Medical Management and Economics. 2014;32(4):263 79.

16. Report of the joint annual review 2016. Matam Medical Region. Available at the Matam medical region on March 25, 2017.

17. Mladovsky P, Ndiaye P, Ndiaye A, Criel B. The impact of stakeholder values and power relations on communitv-based health insurance coverage: qualitative evidence from three Senegalese case studies. Health Policy Plan. 1 Jul 2015;30(6):768 81.

18. Asfaw A, Jütting JP. The Role of Health Insurance in Poverty Reduction: Empirical Evidence from Senegal. International Journal of Public Administration. 2007; 30(8-9):835 58.

19. Aide-mémoire on CMU. Report of the National Agency for Universal Health Coverage. Senegal Ministry of Health and Social Action. [internet] Available November 11, 2016. http://www.sante.gouv.sn/ckfinder/userfiles/files/aidememocmu.pdf.

20. Justin T, Faye S, Nakhimovsky S, Hatt L. Universal Health Coverage Measurement in a Lower-Middle-Income Context: a Senegalese Case Study. Health Finance & Governance Project, Abt Associates Inc. Bethesda, MD; 2014.

21. UEMOA - Regulation No. 07/2010/CM/UEMOA of 1 October 2010 on the status of UEMOA staff (www.droit-afrique.com) - UEMOA-

Reglement-2009-07-mutualite-sociale.pdf [Internet]. [cited 2 Apr 2017]. Available from: http://www.droit-afrique. com/upload/ doc/uemoa/UEMOA-Reglement-2009-07-mutualite-sociale.pdf

22. Microsoft Word - SES-Matam-2013 - SES-Matam-2013.pdf [Internet]. [cited 30 Dec 2016]. Available from: http://www.ansd.sn/ressources/ses/SES- Matam-2013.pdf.

23. Sombié I, Amendah D, Soubeiga KA. Local perceptions of community participation in health in Burkina Faso. Public Health. 5 Nov 2015;27(4):557 64.

24. Séne LM, Cissé M. Catastrophic out-of-pocket payments for health and poverty nexus: evidence from Senegal. Int J Health Econ Manag. 1 Sep 2015;15(3):307 28.

25. Musango L, Dujardin B. Organization and implementation of mutual health insurance: a challenge to the development of health insurance in Rwanda. 28 Jan 2005 [cited 30 Jan 2017]; Available from: http://hdl.handle.net.ezproxy.ulb.ac.be/2013/ULB-DIPOT:oai:dipot.ulb.ac.be:2013/211064.

26. Abiiro GA, Torbica A, Kwalamasa K, et al. Eliciting community preferences for complementary micro health insurance: a discrete choice experiment in rural Malawi. Social Science & Medicine.2014: 120,160-8.

27. Law No. 96-07 of 22 March 1996 transferring powers to the regions, municipalities and rural communities. Law-transfer-region.pdf [Internet].

[cited3May2017]. Available from : http://www.servicepublic.gouv.sn/assets/textes/loi-transfert-region.pdf.

28. Ministry of Health and Social Action of Senegal (2013). Strategic plan for the development of universal health coverage in Senegal 2013-2017. pdf [Internet]. [cited 11 May 2017]. Available from: http://www.coopami.org/fr/countries/countries/senegal/social protection/pdf/soc ial protection05.pdf

29. Chuman, J.; Mulupi, S.; McIntyre, D. Providing financial protection and funding

health service benefits for the informal sector: evidence from sub-Saharan Africa. (2013) 31 pp. GOV.UK [Internet]. [cited 14 May 2017]. Available from: https://www.gov.uk/dfid-research-outputs/providing-financial-protection-and-funding-health-service-benefits-for-the-informal-sector-evidence-from-sub-saharan-africa.

30. Bentein K, Vandenberghe C, Dulac T. Organizational commitment to continuity and indicators of work effectiveness. Revue de gestion des ressources humaines, 2004, vol. 53, p. 69-79.

31. DELOBBE, N. Factors of motivation and transfer training in learning: a sequential study in the context of a leadership training. Factors of motivation and transfer training in learning: a sequential study in the context of a learning. Psychology of Work and Organizations, 2007, vol. 13, no 3, p. 72.

Annexes

Annex 1

Impact of the implementation of the Universal Health Coverage in Senegal : Operational changes as expressed by mutual health insurance stakeholders in the Matam region

Frame

1. Prepare the room for the guest. (Arrangement, quiet place and provide a snack if possible).

2. Introducing yourself to the interviewee

3. Reminder of the theme of the interview, ensure that the subject of the interview is well understood.

4. Agreement to record the interview and specify confidentiality (if possible sign an agreement).

Questions

Presentation

- How would you introduce yourself?
  - Function
  - Length of service
  - Seniority in the position

1. What does your job involve ?

a. How much of your work is directly related to CMU?

b. What is missing in the execution of these tasks?

c. At your level, what is being done to facilitate the execution of the tasks that are devolved to you?

2. How do you perceive the new orientations of the CMU in Senegal?

a. What are the most salient ones?

b. How do you like them?

c. How do they impact your daily work?

3. What are the changes brought about by the CMU that facilitate the work of the mutual insurance company? In terms of :

a. Approval

b. Agreement with the health structures

c. Coverage

d. Cost

i. Membership - subscription

ii. additional payment

iii. relief

iv. co-payment

e. What difficulties do you experience in their execution? Back, reported

4. In your opinion, which priority areas should be focused on the most to improve the current situation of the MOH?

a. Grant

b. Reimbursement

c. Loyalty of the population to mutual health insurance?

d. Other blockages related to the management of MS.

5. What would you recommend globally to ensure the development of mutuals?

a. What is urgent to do?

b. How do you see the future of mutuals in the evolution towards CMU?

<u>**Maintenance fence**</u>

1. Synthesis and feedback: What would you say are the key points to remember from this interview?

2. Do you have anything to add?

3. Could we contact you again for possible clarification.

4. Acknowledgement and see if the interviewee is interested in the results of the study.

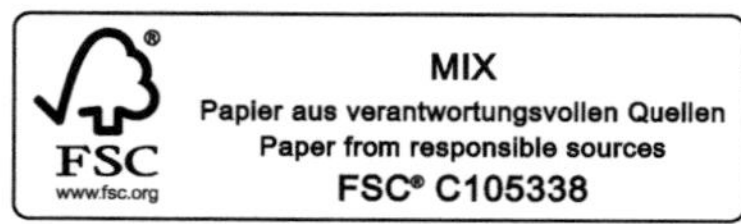

Printed by Books on Demand GmbH, Norderstedt / Germany